Natural Cold and Flu Defense

Using Echinacea, Zinc, Vitamin C and other Supplements/Therapies to Fight Cold and Flu Infection

C.M. Hawken

WOODLAND PUBLISHING
Pleasant Grove, UT

The information in this book is for educational purposes only and is not recommended as a means of diagnosing or treating an illness. All matters concerning physical and mental health should be supervised by a health practitioner knowledgeable in treating that particular condition. Neither the publisher nor author directly or indirectly dispense medical advice, nor do they prescribe any remedies or assume any responsibility for those who choose to treat themselves.

Table of Contents

Colds and Flu:
An Introduction

For many people, the coming of winter months brings the possibility of becoming sick, mainly from colds and the flu. Millions of Americans suffer from at least one bout of the flu or cold each year, resulting in millions of hours of lost work time, millions of dollars spent on "remedy" products, and just plain misery. Those who come down with either end up seeking out syrups, lozenges, tablets and pills that are designed not to eradicate the ailment, but only suppress its various symptoms. To date, there has been no "cure" found for the various strains of viruses that cause colds and flu.

Despite conventional medicine's attempt to suppress the symptoms of the flu and cold, most products remain relatively ineffective and usually bring with them a host of undesired side effects. However, there are natural methods and products that not only help prevent infection from cold and flu viruses, but also help shorten the duration and lessen the severity of a cold/flu infection.

How Do Colds and Flu Differ?

Generally speaking, the differences between a cold and the flu can be imperceptible. However, there are differences. There are more than 20 identified major virus families; most colds come from five of these. Three other virus families produce flu, usually identified as A, B, and C strains. Flu Types B and C are generally mild in adults: both can be confused with bad colds. And once a person has a Type C flu, immunity is usually experienced (though children can get it more than once). The Type A flu virus is the least stable and most volatile when it comes to mutating within the host: it changes its genetic makeup frequently. So, Type A strains cause more severe symptoms than a cold (high fever, extreme fatigue, and a host of respiratory system conditions) and do not usually allow an individual to develop immunity from it. The Type A flu viruses are the viruses of epidemics.

The flu is almost always more severe than a cold, and is usually accompanied by fever, chills and aches. Its onset is also much more rapid than that of a cold. The flu usually lasts anywhere from a few days (there is even strain commonly called the "twenty-four hour flu") to a week. However, residual effects from the bout can last up to a few weeks (this would include fatigue, depression and lack of energy).

Most colds come from one of five virus families, although almost half come from the rhinovirus family. It was only in the late 1980s that the rhinovirus was officially detected. Colds are basically restricted to the nose, throat and surrounding air passages: hence, their official name "upper respiratory tract infection." They usually do not bring fever, chills or the more severe symptoms associated with the flu. But its duration of symptoms is usually longer than that of the flu, sometimes lasting for several weeks at a time.

IS IT THE COLD OR FLU?

SYMPTOMS	COLD	FLU
Fever	Rare	High fever, lasts 3-4 days
Headache	Rare	Prominent
General Aches, Pains	Slight	Usual; often severe
Fatigue, weakness	Quite mild	Can last up to 2-3 weeks
Extreme Fatigue	Never	Early and prominent
Stuffy Nose	Common	Occasionally
Sneezing	Common	Occasionally
Sore Throat	Common	Occasionally
Cough	Mild/moderate	Common; can become severe

The Enemy: Viruses and Bacteria

WHAT ARE VIRUSES AND BACTERIA?

Viruses and bacteria are among this earth's smallest microscopic organisms. Though different in their makeup and activities, they both contribute to the onset of colds and flu. Bacteria, which do not cause colds or flu but can cause secondary conditions, are single-celled beings that abound in our environment—oceans, lakes, air, soil and any moist setting. They are not reliant on an unwilling host for survival, and can survive and reproduce alone. Many bacteria are beneficial to humans, while there are many others that are harmful. These we call pathogenic bacteria, and are those which cause a huge variety of infection and disease to the human body.

Viruses are much smaller than bacteria, measuring anywhere from 1/2 to 1/100th the size of the smallest bacterium. No known viruses are beneficial to the human body. In fact, because viruses are parasites dependent on a host to reproduce and live, they all cause disease to the body. It does this by invading a host cell and commandeering the cell's genetic material as its own, breaking it down and eventually merging with it. In its reproductive processes, the virus ends up destroying the host cell.

All viruses and bacteria can reproduce extremely quickly. Under ideal conditions, one bacterium can reproduce every twenty minutes, which means it could have 16 million "offspring" within a twenty-four hour period. Viruses replicate just as rapidly, which makes clear that when you are fighting a cold or the flu, time is of utmost importance.

HOW DO VIRUSES CAUSE SICKNESS?

Viruses are the cause of the majority of symptoms that accompany a cold or flu. They are involved in the cause of symptoms in several ways. First, some of the symptoms of a cold are caused by the body's own immunological response to the infection; these would include a cough, fever, runny nose, sneezing, watery eyes, etc. Viruses can also prompt what is termed a "disease process," which is the production of antibodies that attach to the viruses they're fighting as both travel throughout the body. Additionally, a virus can destroy or damage vital organs they invade; depending on the extent of the infection in various organs, coupled with the overall virus invasion, the body's immune system can become substantially worn down, making one much more susceptible to other infections.

Fighting The Cold and Flu: How the Immune System Works

This section will be a simplified account of how the body defends itself using various processes and components that are generally classified as the immune system. The body basically uses two interrelated functions—recognition and response—in making its defense mechanisms effective. First, the body is able to recognize foreign agents within the body; these can include anything from a virus to a toxin from cigarette smoke. Once this foreign agent is recognized, the body enlists the help of a variety of cells and molecules to eliminate or neutralize the invader.

To be able to enter the body, the invading organism must first get through physical barriers like the skin and mucous membranes of the nose, throat, and sinuses. These provide an extremely effective barrier to entry by most microorganisms. Intact skin is the most effective barrier; it is compromised when it experiences cuts, scrapes and other wounds. To otherwise gain entry into the body, pathogens must colonize into a formidable number to be able to withstand the various defense cells of the mucous membranes and discharge of mucus by the body to penetrate the mucous membrane. The number of the pathogen must be great enough to withstand the "washing" by saliva, tears, mucous and other fluids, most of which also possess antibacterial and antiviral properties.

If the invading organisms are able to get through the skin and mucous membranes, there are several other immune system barriers waiting. The body's temperature is an effective deterrent to many organisms. For instance, anthrax, a serious condition common to many farm animals, does not affect chickens because of the chickens' high body temperature. Hydrochloric acid, found in the stomach, is also a major barrier to infection. Very few viruses that make it past the mucous membranes of the nose and throat to the stomach can survive the stomach's acid and low pH. Interferon is another of the body's great immunity agents. It is derived from virus infected cells, thereby enabling it to bind with and neutralize nearby virus cells; if there is enough of the interferon, it can neutralize large numbers of the invading virus.

THE BODY'S FIGHTER CELLS

There are two major groups of phagocytes (any cell that destroys foreign particles) in the immune system: antigen producing cells, called B-lymphocytes, and which mature within bone marrow; and T-cells, which are produced by the thymus gland. These antigen producers are supported by the other glands in the body (otherwise known as the lymphoid organs), which include the lymph nodes, spleen, and mucosal associated lymphoid tissue, and the tonsils, appendix and Peyer's patches. One of the fantastic aspects of these "producers" is their ability to take over the production of antigens by another immobilized producer. The following gives a brief description of the body's fighter cells and their functions.

B Cells: These mature in the bone marrow and produce antibodies to inhibit activity of foreign agents. B cells account for 10-15 percent of all lymphocytes.

T Cells: These mature in the thymus gland and direct their activity against specific invading antigens (such as a specific flu strain). They make up about 75 percent of the body's lymphocytes.

Helper T Cells: These cells, also known as T-4 cells, are a specific type of T cell that secrete the proteins interleukin and interferon to stimulate B cells and Killer T cells. They make up a large portion of all T cells.

Killer T Cells: Also known as T-8 cells, these bind themselves to a specific invading cell and inject it with enzymes that aid in destroying it. Killer T cells make up about 25 percent of all T cells.

Suppressor T Cells: These cells act to prevent excessive immune response by the body; they can actually suppress the activity of the other lymphocytes.

Natural Killer Cells: These cells are nonspecific (neither B nor T cells), free-ranging cells that can recognize and kill any invading cell on first contact. They are the body's most potent weapon, possessing over 100 biochemical "poisons" for destroying invading cells. Natural killer cells account for only 5-10 percent of the body's lymphocytes.

Prevention—The Best Medicine

Since there are no known "cures" for colds or flu, prevention is often the best medicine. In fact, taking preventive measures against the cold and flu will also improve your overall health. The following areas provide prevention tips in various areas.

HYGIENE

Wash Your Hands

This is a simple, yet extremely effective way to avoid flu or cold infection. Most cold and flu viruses are spread by direct contact and "self-inoculation" (making yourself sick by touching a virus-contaminated object or person, then touching your mouth, nose or eyes). Evidence shows this is all it takes for you to become infected. Wash often during the day, especially if you are around sick people. Washing with soap (antibacterial soaps are good disinfectants) or just plain hot water are great virus deterrents.

Avoid Touching Your Face

Because cold and flu viruses enter through the mouth, nose and eyes, touching one's face is a risky practice when trying to avoid becoming sick. Studies have shown that most adults, whether conscientiously or not, touch their face more than fifteen times an hour. A concentrated effort to avoid this can greatly decrease the risk of catching a cold or the flu.

Keep a Sick Room (or house) Healthy

If there is someone in the home who is sick, make sure to keep their room, and the whole house, well sanitized. The following guidelines will aid you in doing this:

• Change and wash their bed linens daily.
• Wipe with disinfectant all lamp and light switches, telephones, door knobs, TV remote controls, or anything else the infected person might touch.
• Periodically air out room by opening doors and windows. Continually introducing fresh air reduces the risk of other persons in the house becoming infected.

DIET AND NUTRITION

Eat Healthful Foods

Eating right will not only help prevent virus infections, but will also help promote overall good health. Healthful eating habits encourage healthy cell and tissue reproduction, maintain strong bone and tissues, provide the necessary nutrients for the immune system to operate at top levels, and allow the body to run efficiently and avoid unnecessary stress. Ensure that your diet follows the guidelines given by the FDA , namely the "Food Pyramid." This pyramid outlines the different food groups and the approximate servings one should eat daily to encourage good levels of health.

It is important to remember that there are several factors that determine how one should eat. Age is one of these. For example, most young to middle age adults should consume about 2,000 calories. This number decreases, however, once you are over fifty. The older you are, the "smarter" you must eat. Metabolism slows with age, as does the body's ability to effectively utilize nutrients. Studies show that as one's age increases, so does their risk of contracting more severe strains of the flu and cold.

Probably one of the most sound pieces of advice when determining what and how to eat is that of eating "whole" foods; that is, foods that are in their basic, or natural, state. These would include fresh fruits and vegetables, nuts, and whole grains. Of course, dishes including any of these would generally be considered healthful. Whole foods contain "phytonutrients," compounds such as flavonoids, essential fatty acids, and antioxidants that protect the body and provide the necessary elements for optimal function. As foods are broken down more and more (e.g., processed, cooked, synthesized), their most valuable components are often lost. One cannot overestimate the importance of a healthful diet in not only preventing the onset of colds and flu, but of achieving overall good health.

Drink Plenty of Fluids

Because nearly seventy-five percent of the body is water, and because water is necessary for most of the body's defense functions, it is very important to keep the body's fluid level's at optimum levels. A typical adult needs eight 8-ounce glasses of water or clear liquids a day. Schedule breaks throughout your day to make sure you receive adequate fluids.

Exercise

Exercise is essential for overall good health. Aerobic exercise is especially beneficial; it speeds up the heart to pump larger quantities of blood; makes you breathe heavier and faster to aid in the oxygen transfer from the lungs to the cardiovascular system; and forces your body to flush out toxins through sweat once the body's temperature rises. Eventually, aerobic exercise forces the body's cells to use larger amounts of the blood's oxygen, making those body tissues more healthy and able to defend themselves.

Exercise also helps the body by relieving stress; it gets rid of excess adrenaline, triggers the release of endorphins, which helps relieve depression, and strengthens muscles, bones and body tissues. Studies also show that the body's immune system is directly aided by exercise because of the increased release of the body's virus-killing cells.

Basically, exercise is very beneficial for the body's overall health, and can help prevent infection by a cold or flu virus. It doesn't matter what kind of exercise you do; the important thing is that you do it.

OTHER RECOMMENDATIONS

Avoid Smoking

Smoking does several things to not only promote the onset of colds and flu, but to encourage more severe ones. Smoking dries the cilia in the mucous membranes, paralyzing them in their ability to trap and sweep out viruses. Smoking also introduces an overload of toxins to the mucous membranes, making it nearly impossible for the cilia that aren't disabled to get rid of these toxins and any other pathogens (cold and flu viruses included). There is an overwhelming mountain of evidence pointing to a direct link between smoking and all forms of respiratory ailments.

Avoid Consuming Alcohol

Alcohol is a depressant that slows body responses to the environment, including that of eliminating cold and flu viruses. As most people know, heavy alcohol consumption destroys the liver, one the main organs involved in cleaning and filtering the body of unwanted toxins. Alcohol also depletes mineral and vitamin stores and is dehydrating to the body, further diminishing the body's ability to battle the onset of flu or colds.

Get Plenty of Rest

The importance of sleep and rest in optimizing the body's ability to fight infection cannot be overemphasized. Numerous studies show that Americans in general do not get enough good quality sleep. Sleep is the time the body is at its best in cleaning the body of unwanted materials, repairing damaged cells, supplying nutrients and essentially revitalizing the body.

Reduce Stress

Stress is one of the most common factors contributing to the onset of colds and flu. While stress is a natural part of life, it can sometimes overwhelm a person. There is much research indicating that effective stress management not only helps prevent the onset of various diseases, but also shortens their duration. Identifying and coping with sources of stress can certainly help maintain a healthy immune system.

SHOULD I REALLY TAKE THAT COLD MEDICINE?

Americans spend literally billions of dollars each year on the hundreds of available nonprescription cold and flu medicines. These medicines are usually designed to rid specific symptoms of the cold and flu, rather than attacking the actual virus causing the symptoms. There are several types of medications: analgesics, antihistamines, decongestants and cough remedies, among others.

While sometimes it may seem beneficial to treat a specific symptom, there is something very important to remember. Cold or flu symptoms (such as coughing, runny nose or fever) are usually mechanisms employed by the body to effectively rid itself of the invading virus. For instance, the body may make its temperature rise to fever levels because the higher temperatures can actually kill a virus (the optimal temperature for survival of most viruses is 85 degrees, so a temperature of 101 degrees would seem a good way to get rid of the virus). Many experts agree that the symptoms are a necessary part of the healing process. Enduring the temporary discomfort of some of the symptoms may actually let the body to deal more effectively with the virus and allow the virus to more rapidly run its course.

So why not take conventional cold medications? Well, if coughing is one of the ways the body rids itself of the viruses trapped in mucus, then how is it beneficial to suppress the cough and thereby allow the viruses to remain in the respiratory system? There is an impressive body of research indicating that many cough, cold and flu medicines not only suppress the necessary "symptoms" of the cold and flu, but also depress the immune system as well.

Natural Treatments for Preventing and Treating Colds and Flu

Natural treatments for the cold and flu can include a variety of things from eating chicken soup to using humidifiers. It is also well-known that certain nutrients, specifically vitamins and minerals and other herbal/natural substances, have a large impact on how our immune system functions. The following quote, taken from a study in a respected nutritional journal, demonstrates just how important these nutrients can be:

"Nutrition and nutritional status can have a profound effects on immune functions, resistance to infection and autoimmunity in man and other animals. Nutrients enhance or depress immune function depending on the nutrient and level of its intake. Protein-energy malnutrition and vitamin A deficiency are strongly associated with impaired immunity and infectious disease. The essential role vitamin A plays in infection and maintenance of mucosal surfaces has long been known. Recent evidence shows that T-cell subpopulations, cytokines and antibody subclasses are all affected by vitamin A. In animal studies, supplementation with vitamin E protects against infection and is linked to stimulatory effects on the immune system. In man, vitamin E and other antioxidants increase the number of CD4+ cells. Dietary lipids and zinc have a substantial impact on autoimmunity from protective to potentiation of immuno-pathological processes in animals. Dietary copper is important in the prevention of infection in some animal species and T-cell function is defective under deficiency states due to an inability to produce IL-2. Selenium has been linked to viral infection, enhanced T-cell functions and TNF beta induced increase in natural killer cell activity. Understanding the molecular and cellular immunological mechanisms involved in nutrient-immune interactions will increase our applications for nutrition of the immune system in health and in disease" (Harbige, L.S. 285-86).

Herbal/Natural Supplements for Treating Cold/Flu Infection

ECHINACEA

Concerning the maintenance and strengthening of the immune system, echinacea is one of the most well-known and respected. The various echinacea species (*E. angustifolia, E. purpurea,* and *E. pallida* are the most commonly used) have yielded an impressive array of chemical constituents possessing pharmacological properties. This would suggest that there is some sort of synergistic action between the compounds to achieve the therapeutic benefits. Echinacea's major constituents with therapeutic properties are polysaccharides, flavonoids, caffeic acid derivatives, essential oils, polyacetylenes, and alkylamides. As stated previously, these constituents are responsible for a number of immunostimulatory, anti-inflammatory, antiviral, antibacterial and anticancer properties (Murray, 93). The following gives a brief overview of echinacea's various benefits, and how they relate specifically to preventing and treating the cold and flu.

Echinacea and the Immune System

Echinacea exerts several effects on the immune system. One of these influences what is called the alternate complement pathway, which enhances the movement of white blood cells into the areas of infection. Inulin, one of echinacea's most highly regarded compounds, is thought to be responsible for this. Echinacea is also thought to increase the production of properdin, a serum protein that also enhances the activity of the alternate complement pathway (Murray, 97).

Echinacea also affects many of the immune systems various cells responsible for retarding viral and bacterial infection. For instance, it is known to stimulate the activity of the body's T-cells, or lymphocytes, resulting in more production of interferon. These T-cells are also responsible for what is called "cell-mediated immunity." Dr. Michael Murray, a well-respected naturopathic physician, explains, "Cell-mediated immunity refers to immune mechanisms not controlled or mediated by antibodies. Cell-mediated immunity is extremely important in providing resistance to infection by moldlike bacteria, yeast, fungi, parasites, and viruses" (98). These T-cells are also responsible for activating the "natural killer cells," the body's first line of defense against cancer development and instrumental in protecting against cold and flu viruses.

Echinacea has also been shown to enhance the performance of the immune system's macrophages, the cells that essentially "eat" or engulf foreign material, including bacteria, viruses, and dead cellular matter.

Echinacea's Antiviral Properties

It is known that the aerial portion of *E. purpurea,* as well as extracts of its root, is effective in warding off viruses. Studies have demonstrated that echinacea inhibits various types of viruses, including the influenza (flu), herpes and vesicular stomatitis virus (Murray, 99). How does echinacea work when fighting the onset of virus infection? It is known to block virus receptors on the cell surface, but its most significant action may be that of inhibiting the viruses production of hyaluronidase, the enzyme responsible for allowing virus cells to spread and become more invasive. Echinacea's ability to restrict hyaluronidase production is probably its most impressive antiviral capability.

Echinacea is also able to "kill" viruses indirectly by encouraging the production and release of interferon, the substance capable of blocking the transcription of viral RNA (and thereby blocking its reproduction).

There are numerous studies supporting echinacea's ability to fight colds and flu. A 1992 study targeted more than 100 patients suffering from cold symptoms. The study lasted eight weeks: half of the patients received echinacea supplements, and the other half received a placebo. The results were impressive: 35 percent of those receiving the echinacea remained healthy the entire eight weeks, compared to only 25 percent of the placebo group. The length of time between infections for the echinacea was nearly 40 percent longer than that of the placebo group. And infections occurring in patients receiving echinacea were of shorter duration and significantly less severe (Schoneberger 2-12).

ZINC

Zinc has long been recognized in natural health circles for providing protection against colds. However, it has only been recently that the rest of the population has been exposed to its cold-fighting abilities. It is well known that zinc deficiencies are linked to immune system-related disorders and the increased susceptibility to infectious diseases.

Over the last few years, zinc throat lozenges have become very popular in treating colds. There has been much debate as to whether they actually worked or not. There is now a significant amount of research concerning zinc lozenge products showing that they are effective; they not only help prevent the onset of colds, but also cause a notable decrease in a cold's duration. One such study states: "A randomized, double-blind, placebo-controlled clinical trial has shown that treatment of the common cold with zinc gluconate lozenges resulted in a significant reduction in duration of symptoms of the cold. Patients received zinc-containing lozenges or placebo lozenges every 2 hours for the duration of cold symptoms. The median time to complete resolution of cold symptoms was 4.4 days in the zinc group compared with 7.6 days in the placebo group" (*Nutr.-Rev,* 82-3).

Another recent study clearly shows that zinc is not only beneficial to the immune system, but necessary for its optimal function. The report focused on infants with zinc deficiencies who showed characteristic skin rash, alopecia, retarded growth, generalized edema and decreased serum alkaline phosphatase. After adding zinc supplementation to the infants' diet, the symptoms greatly decreased. "A high dose of elemental zinc (2.5 mg/kg/day), administered orally, improved the clinical symptoms and restored the immune function. In patients with zinc deficiency, impaired neutrophil adhesion and lymphocyte function may contribute to immunodeficiency which can be reversed with adequate zinc supplementation" (Fan, et al. 364).

VITAMIN C

One of the most well-known nutrients for battling the effects of colds and flu is vitamin C. For years (largely due to Dr. Linus Pauling's research on the vitamin), its benefits have been known. There is a large body of research that indicates that it is effective in reducing the severity and duration of colds and flu. Additionally, beyond its antiviral and antibacterial properties, vitamin C acts as an immunostimulant. It enhances white blood cell production, increases interferon (a group of proteins released by white blood cells that combat a virus) levels and antibody responses, promotes secretion of thymic hormones, and improves connective tissue. These important capabilities can't be overlooked, say Shari Lieberman and Nancy Bruning, authors of *The Real Vitamin and Mineral Book*:

> "Despite media hype, though, most people don't realize just how many important functions are performed by this nutrient. . . . Perhaps foremost among vitamin C's many functions is the major role it plays in the immune system, where, according to growing evidence, it helps increase resistance to a range of diseases, including infections and cancer. Ascorbic acid appears to be required by the thymus gland (one of the major glands involved in immunity), and increases the mobility of the phagocytes, the type of cell that "eats" bacteria, viral cells, and cancer cells, as well as other harmful foreign invaders" (121)

Of special note is the necessity of vitamin C for elderly individuals. An increase in age usually brings a decrease in immune system function, thereby allowing for greater risk of infection and disease. Studies have shown that supplementation with vitamin C results in significant improvement in immune function in elderly persons.

How much vitamin C should one take? There is conflicting information on this, however, most experts agree that the recommended intake suggested by the FDA (60 mg) is not sufficient. In fact, Lieberman and Bruning suggest, "An optimum intake for humans may be 1,000 milligrams or more daily—an amount far higher than the RDI of 60 milligrams" (126). Many doctors also suggest taking large doses—as much as 10,000 mg—while suffering from a cold or flu.

One of the great things about vitamin C is that it is found abundantly in various fruits and vegetables—this lends to its being consumed in acceptable amounts without having to take supplements. The best food sources include broccoli, sweet peppers, collards, cabbage, spinach, kale, parsley, melons, potatoes, tangerines and Brussels sprouts. Of course, there are many other foods that are excellent sources of vitamin C.

GARLIC

Garlic (*Allium sativum*), whose culinary prowess is extremely well known, is one of the most commonly used medicinal herbs, found throughout the world and having been employed for various therapeutic purposes for thousands of years. It is common in Chinese herbal medicine, ayurvedic medicine, and has recently received much attention from mainstream news media in the U.S. and other Western countries. Recent research indicates that it possesses some powerful capabilities relating to the immune system and the body's ability to fight infection.

So, how does garlic aid the body in fighting viral infection? Like other herbal and natural substances, garlic possesses antiviral and antibacterial capabilities and has been shown repeatedly to stimulate and improve performance by the body's immune systems. First and foremost, garlic has been shown to kill viruses; for the purposes of this booklet, the viruses shown to succumb to garlic's antiviral action include the common cold and flu viruses.

The major weakness of conventional antibiotics is that they are not effective at all in treating viral infections; in other words, they will not work against cold or flu viruses. They also don't work against more serious viral infections, such as viral meningitis, viral pneumonia, or herpes. Multiple studies on garlic pinpoint its ability to actually ward off, or kill, flu and cold viruses (Bergner 105-6).

Besides having a direct effect on cold and flu viruses, garlic can also protect the body from invading virus cells by enhancing the body's immune functions. For instance, several of garlic's chemical constituents, including allicin and diallyl trisulfide, have been shown in studies to activate the body's natural killer cells and macrophages, increase B-cell activity and increase the production of antibodies (Bergner 109-110). All this equates to improved chances of resisting infection by invading cold and flu viruses. The following is a list of the most prominent viruses, bacteria, and other microbes inhibited by garlic: *Candida albicans, Cryptosporidium, Escherichia coli, Herpes simplex* virus types 1 and 2, human rhinovirus type 2, influenza B, *Mycobacterium tuberculosis, Parainfluenza* virus type 3, and *Streptococcus faecalis* (Bergner 101).

GOLDENSEAL

Goldenseal (*Hydrastis canadensis*), which is native to North America, was used extensively by Native American tribes for a wide variety of ailments, including infections. It is currently a favorite among herbalists for its proven therapeutic capabilities. The pharmacological activity of the plant is attributed mainly to three alkaloids: canadine, hydrastine and berberine. There is substantial research to back up these alkaloids' effect on various bacteria and viruses. Berberine, for instance, has demonstrated the ability to inhibit the activity of *Staphylococcus spp., Streptococcus, spp., Chlamydia spp.,* and *Salmonella typhi,* and is recognized as the plant's most valuable constituent.

Another reason goldenseal is effective in combating invasion of colds and flu is that of its ability to stimulate the immune system. Berberine stimulates the activity of macrophages, one of the body's defense mechanisms directly responsible for destroying invading viruses, bacteria, cancer cells and other "invaders." Berberine has also been shown to enhance blood flow to the spleen, which has several responsibilities in aiding the body's immune responses (Murray, Pizzorno 67).

Besides goldenseal's ability to directly fight bacteria/viruses and stimulate the immune system, it also is useful in maintaining healthy mucous membranes. It heals irritated membranes, which is one of the most annoying of all symptoms brought on by cold or flu; it also strengthens the mucous linings, making them less susceptible to irritation by cold/flu infection; the herb's hydrastine content has also been shown to be an effective anti-inflammatory, which can worsen symptoms of cold and flu infection. Not surprising is the notion that goldenseal is one of the most requested herbal remedies during the winter months.

PAU D'ARCO

Pau d'arco (*Tabebuia avellanedae*), also known as "taheebo" and "lapacho," is another herbal supplement known for its powerful antiviral, antibiotic and immune system enhancing capabilities. Pau d'arco is not an herb in the typical sense; it is the inner bark of the *Tabebuia avellanedae* tree (which can grow upwards of 120 feet) that is widely used for its medicinal properties. Though its principal use is not for treating an already established bout of cold or flu, it is very effective in strengthening the immune system, thereby preventing the onset of viral infection.

Pau d'arco is one of the most widely researched herbal products of the Western Hemisphere, though its therapeutic applications remain relatively obscure when compared with herbal supplements such as aloe vera, garlic, or ginseng. The research that has been done (most of it conducted in South American countries of Argentina, Brazil, Paraguay, where the tree grows) is impressive; the tree's bark contains several key compounds, among them lapachol, a napthoquinone, which are known to possess the powerful antiviral, antibiotic and anticancer effects. The bark is also used as an anti-inflammatory, which would make it useful for symptoms of cold and flu infection.

This body of research is impressive; there are literally dozens of studies indicating that the herb is effective in enhancing the performance of the immune system, in fighting a wide variety of viruses, bacteria and parasites, and in inhibiting the activity of cancerous cells. In fact, the anticancer effects of lapachol were studied by the National Cancer Institute, beginning in 1968.

Pau d'Arco's Antiviral Properties

Lapachol, beta-lapachone, hydroxynapthoquinone and other constituents have been shown to actively inhibit the activity of several viruses, including both herpes viruses (I and II), the influenza viruses, polioviruses and vesicular stomatitis virus. (Linhares and De Santana, Lagrota, et al., and Selway). In *The Healing Power of Herbs,* Dr. Michael Murray says concerning beta-lapachone's antiviral activity: "Studies of beta-lapachone's antiviral activity have offered insights into the mechanism of this powerful quinone. In experiments with viruses, beta-lapachone demonstrated its ability to inhibit certain key viral enzymes, such as DNA and RNA polymerases, and retrovirus reverse transcriptase. These actions have great significance in the possible treatment of acquired immunodeficiency syndrome (AIDS), Epstein-Barr virus, and other viral infections" (223).

How to Take Pau d'Arco

Michael Murray notes that the most popular way of taking pau d'arco is in that of a decoction. The standard dose of the decoction is about one cup of decocted bark two to eight times daily. The decoction can be made by boiling one teaspoon of pau d'arco for each cup of water for five to fifteen minutes. Another popular way of administering the herb is through a steeping the bark to make tea.

There has been conflicting reports of how potent the bark can be. This is certainly understandable, since there are undoubtedly products on the market that vary in their way of harvesting, the maturity of bark harvested, and the actual type of tree from which the bark was harvested (there are other trees in the *Tabebuia* genus that are generally included as part of the pau d'arco family). Make sure you buy only from reputable sources—this will ensure a higher quality product.

ASTRAGALUS

Astragalus (*Astragalus membranaceus*) is extremely popular in Chinese herbal medicine, where it is employed for a wide variety of ailments. It is recognized by Chinese herbalists as an immune system enhancer. But its reputation is not limited to just folk use. There have been clinical trials conducted, most of them in China, that have demonstrated that both the severity and length of the common cold are reduced by application of astragalus (Chang, But 1041-46).

LICORICE

Licorice (*Glycyrriza glabra*) is popular in many herbal cold/flu products for its immune enhancing abilities, and its effect on various cold/flu symptoms, including coughing and congestion. Modern research backs the historical use, showing licorice to have the ability to fight viruses and bacteria, and to stimulate the immune system.

PEPPERMINT (AND OTHER MINTS)

The mint family is extremely popular in herbal medicine. The different varieties have been used for a myriad of disorders for hundreds of years. The menthol contained in peppermint and other mint plants is helpful in treating various cold and flu symptoms, especially that of soothing irritated throat, sinuses and skin (lips, nose). It can be used in ointments, salves, lozenges, inhalants and decongestants. Clincal studies have also shown the mint family to demonstrate some antiviral capabilities (especially when taken in tea form).

BETA CAROTENE (VITAMIN A)

Vitamin A (and its precursor beta carotene) has long been known to be effective against infectious diseases, including the common cold and the various flu strains. It has antiviral and antibacterial capabilities. A deficiency of vitamin A can manifest itself through increased infection by cold/flu viruses.

Other Natural Therapies for Treating Colds and Flu

HOMEOPATHY

Homeopathic remedies have long been recognized for treating colds and flu. Many believers of homeopathy are now mixing the modern practice of injection with homeopathy, introducing the remedy via injection into a muscle or intravenously

(*Alternative Medicine* 636). There are several homeopathic remedies effective against the cold and flu:

*Allium cepa:*For those with thin, burning discharge from the eyes and nose and who sneeze frequently

*Nux vomica:*For those who have a runny nose during the day and have nasal congestion during the night. These individuals may also be impatient and irritable.

Aconitum napellus: For those who experience sudden cold or flu symptoms that begin only after being exposed to significant cold. This individual may feel better in open air, yet worse after midnight.

Natrum muriaticum: For the individual with a substantial watery nasal discharge. Other symptoms include sneezing, lost of taste and smell, and constant thirst.

Other commonly used homeopathic remedies for cold and flu symptoms include *Eupatorium perfoliatum, Belladonna,* and *Baptisia.*

HYDROTHERAPY

Hydrotherapy consisting of sudden shifts from hot to cold water temperatures can help the body become accustomed to shifts in temperature, climate and humidity. This is because many outbreaks of flu and cold often coincide with dramatic changes in season and temperature. If done consistently, this "contrast" hydrotherapy can be as simple as running the last minute of a shower at a colder temperature (*Alternative Medicine* 637).

Conclusion

When considering how to combat the onset of a cold or the flu, there are several therapies and natural products that aid the body in not only preventing, but also effectively eliminating the invading virus. Prevention is usually thought of as the best medicine; healthful eating habits, nutrient supplementation, exercise, and good hygiene can prevent viral infection. And in case of contracting a cold/flu virus, there are herbal and other natural products that can effectively lessen the severity of and reduce the length of any bout of flu or cold. Preventing and "curing" the onset of cold and flu may not be as difficult as once thought.

Bibliography

Bergner, Paul. *The Healing Power of Garlic.* Rocklin, California: Prima Publishing, 1996.

Burton Goldberg Group. *Alternative Medicine: The Definitive Guide.* Fife, Washington: Future Medicine Publishing, 1997.

Chang, H.M. and But, P.P.H. *Pharmacology and Applications of Chinese Materia Medica, vol. 2.* World Scientific Publishing, Teaneck, NJ: 1987, 1041-46.

Lagrota, M., et al. "Antiviral Activity of Lapachol." *Review of Microbiology* 14 (1983): 21-26.

Lieberman, Shari, PhD, Nancy Bruning. *The Real Vitamin and Mineral Book.* Garden City Park, New York: Avery Publishing Group, 1997.

Linhares, M. and De Santana C.F. "Estudo sobre of efeito de substancias antibioticas obtidas de Streptomyces e vegetais superiores sobre o herpevirus hominis. *Revista Instituto Antibioticos, Recife* 15 (1975): 25-32.

Murray, Michael T. *The Healing Power of Herbs.* Rocklin, Ca.: Prima, 1995.

Murray, Michael, N.D., and Joseph Pizzorno, N.D. *Encyclopedia of Natural Medicine.* Rocklin, California: Prima Publishing, 1991.

Schoneberger, D. "The Influence of Immune-Stimulating Effects of Pressed Juice from Echinacea purpurea on the Course and Severity of Colds." *Forum of Immunology* (8)1992: 2-12.

Selway, J. "Antiviral Activity of Flavones and Flavins." In: *Plant Flavonoids in Biology and Medicine: Biochemical, Pharmacological, and Structure-Activity Relationships.* New York: Alan R. Liss, 1986: 521-536.